LAPAROSCOPIC TOTAL EXTRA - PERITONEAL GROIN HERNIA REPAIR TECHNIQUE USING BALLOON

Groin Hernia Surgery option without going inside patient Abdomen (Tummy).

SSabri

Table of Contents

Preface 1
Introduction...2,3
Modalities of Surgical Treatment... 4
Understanding Abdominal Wall Anatomy 5
What is TEP Repair? 6,7,8,9
Port Position for TEP Repair 10
Port Placement Technique 11,12
Hernia Anatomy for Surgeons and Patient Awareness ...13,14
Mesh Trimming Technique.. 15
Use of Glue to Secure the Mesh in Peritoneal Space 16,17
Complications of TEP Repair 18,19,20
Patient Questions.. 21
References.. 22

Preface

Groin hernia is a common surgical condition. It involves both planned and emergency surgery. In terms of elective surgery open and laparoscopic, robotic surgeries are the options. Elective surgery can be performed with a Total extra-peritoneal approach without entering inside the patient's abdomen. Peritoneum is a sheath of smooth tissue that lines the abdominal cavity and surrounds the abdominal organs. It pads and insulates the organs and secretes lubricating fluid to reduce the friction.

My work is part of patient education series to create awareness and remove the scientific jargon for an easy understanding of condition. TEP surgery advantages are in unilateral or bilateral hernia, following previous open hernia repair, previous abdominal surgical history including lower midline incision.

Work is dedicated to the loving memory of my deceased dad and girl's grandad (A K Sabri). He was a passionate lover of making BBQ in his free time. He himself underwent groin hernia surgery in his lifetime.

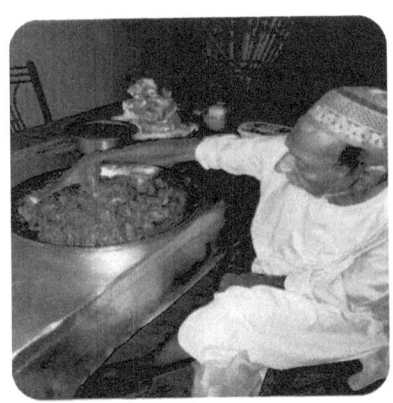

Special Thanks
Mohammad Aamir, Areej, Areeb.

Introduction

Hernia

- **Epidemiology and Incidence**

Abdominal wall hernia is a common pathology that affects 1.7% of the entire population over their lifetime. It is estimated that over 20 million abdominal wall hernias are repaired worldwide every year.

- **How people develop hernia**

Hernia develops through a weakness in muscle or surrounding tissues. Hernia may present at birth called congenital hernia or develop at a later part of a person's life. In my description I am concentrating only on inguinal and femoral variety and TEP repair approach. On lying down the hernia lump usually drops back and there is often nothing to feel. TEP approach is suitable for non-obstructed / non incarcerated hernia. Majority of hernia gets bigger if not treated electively and there is risk of obstruction and strangulation in them.

- **Inguinal hernia**

It's one of the most common types of hernia it mainly affects men. The defect is in the top inner part of the thigh. If a hernia is confirmed clinically, usually no further investigations are required except in co-morbid patients. Although there are options of Ultrasound, Ct scan, MRI scan available with diagnostic difficulties.

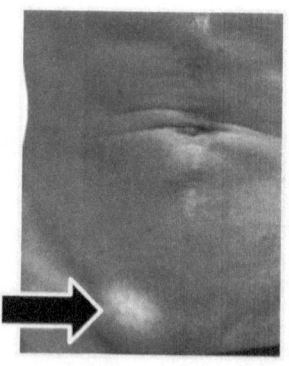

Groin hernia presents as a lump above and medial to pubic tubercle

- **Femoral Hernia**

Femoral hernia makes up 5-10 % of all hernia, they are more common in females. Old age, and muscle weakness contribute to its development. TEP repair is a suitable option for a non-obstructed variety of hernia.

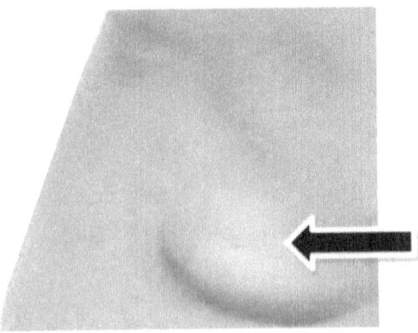

Femoral hernia in right groin below and lateral to pubic tubercle

Modalities of surgical treatment

- Traditionally, open procedures were performed for all types of hernia, but since 1990s minimally invasive procedures were developed to treat this condition. Now a days, these encompass both laparoscopic and robotic hernia repair procedures.

- When discussing about minimally invasive surgical treatment of abdominal wall hernias, two types of techniques have been widely deployed: intra-peritoneal procedures (TAPP – Transabdominal pre-peritoneal) and extra-peritoneal (TEP/E - TEP - totally extra- peritoneal or extended totally extra-peritoneal).

Understanding Abdominal wall Anatomy

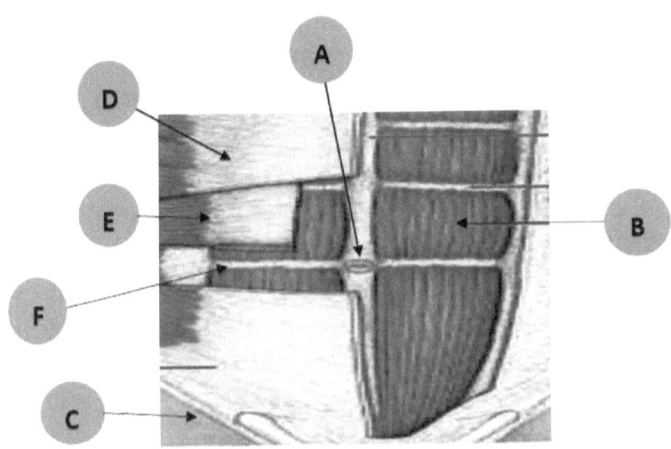

Abdominal wall anatomy in relation to TEP hernia repair

- Umbilicus (A)
- Rectus Abdominis (B)
- Inguinal Ligament (C)
- External Oblique (D)
- Internal Oblique (E)
- Transversus Abdominis (F)

What is TEP REPAIR?

- TEP is a recognized technique for inguinal hernia repair involving usually three small skin incisions as per picture, followed by blunt subcutaneous fat dissection and incision of anterior rectus sheath with lateral retraction of muscles.

- Blunt dissection is performed in the preperitoneal space, facilitated by the "balloon dissector" which is introduced in this space. The operation is performed without entering the abdominal cavity and hence less chances of injury to the intraperitoneal organs and/or future adhesions.

- A mesh is used in the extra-peritoneal space to protect the hernia orifice, following reduction of herniated organs. The procedure is performed under general anesthetic, as day surgery. The average duration of a unilateral inguinal hernia repair by TEP procedure is around 60 mins. This is similar to a TAPP groin hernia repair.

- The main advantage of this technique is reduced post operative pain due to smooth tissue dissection facilitated by "spacer" instrument with consecutive shorter post operative recovery time and reduced length of stay, altogether with avoidance of intra-peritoneal entry and theoretically minimizing risks of intra-peritoneal organs injury and intra-peritoneal adhesion.

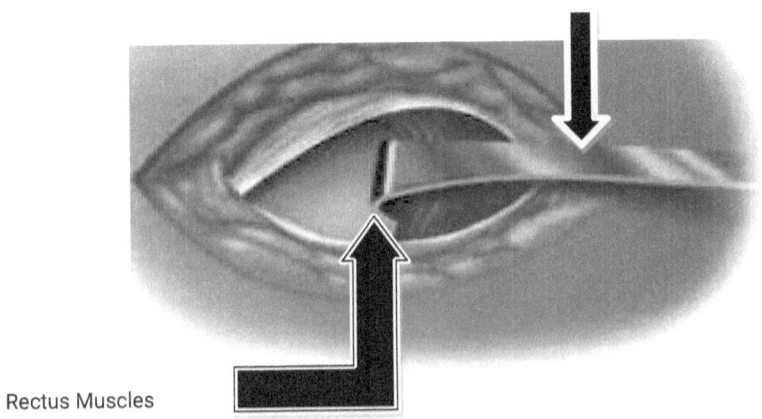

Pre-peritoneal is created after dissection of rectus muscles.

In TEP approach, after dividing the anterior rectus sheath, rectus muscle are splitted up to create the space using balloon. Langenbeck retractor to split up the muscle after dividing the anterior rectus sheath. Balloon in preperitoneal space to be inflated to create the space advancing towards the pubic bone. Laparoscopic Balloon is used above the peritoneum to create space for dissection.

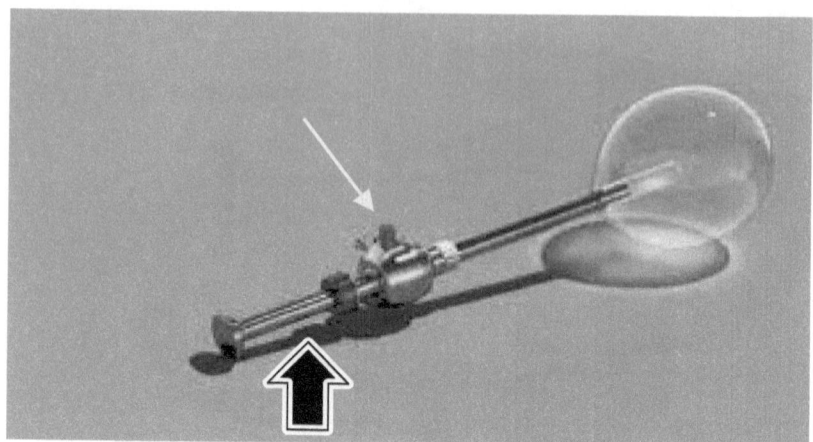

- Laparoscopic Balloon are plastic or metal.

- Blunt trocars are used to create the preperitoneal space.

- Yellow arrow pointing towards air insufflation mechanism, Inner tubing of trocar.

- Black arrow showing the metallic tube.

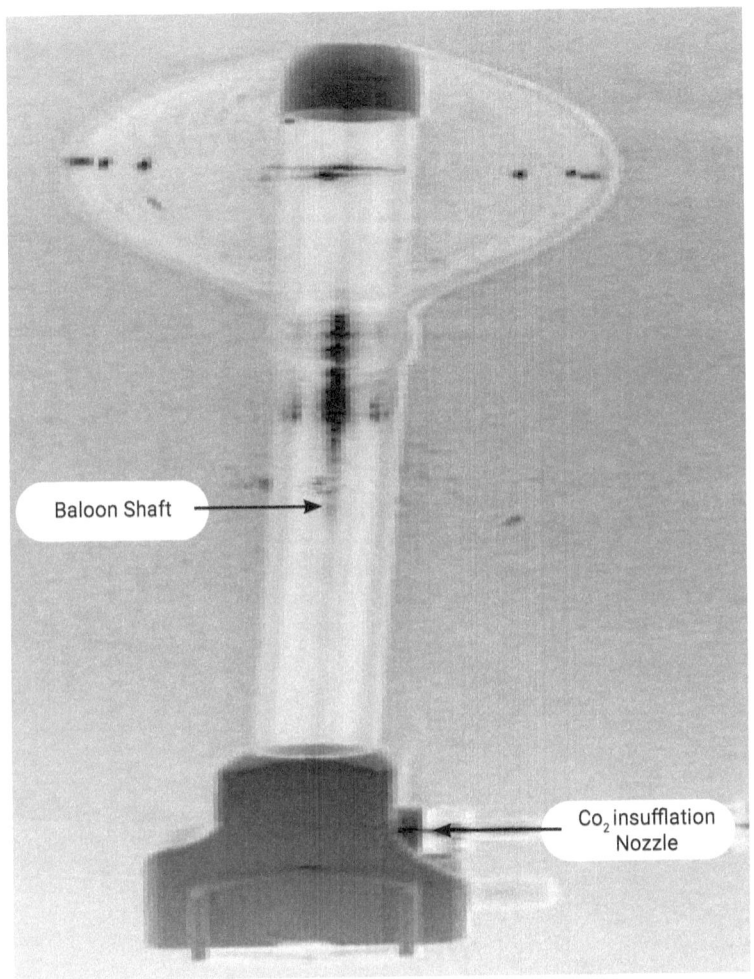

Plastic balloon to inflate and create the preperitoneal space

Port Position for TEP Repair

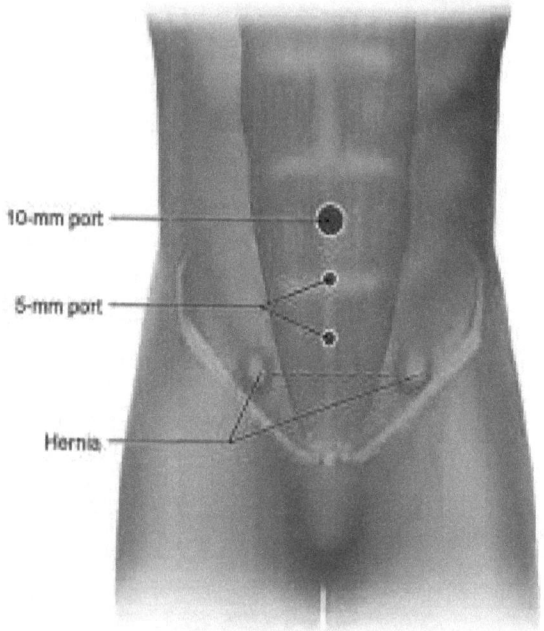

3 ports are placed for TEP surgery including a 10 mm port for umbilical area and 2 (5 mm) ports below it for dissection purposes. The lowest port is 2-3 cm above pubic symphysis and 3rd (5 mm) port is placed between the two ports.

Port Placement Technique

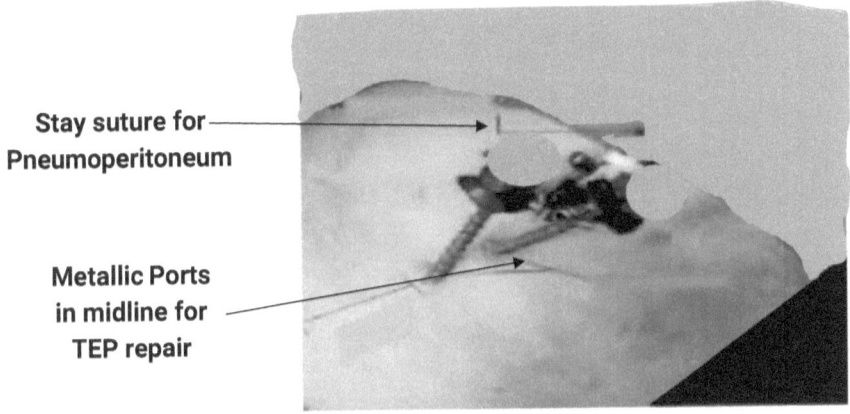

Stay suture for Pneumoperitoneum

Metallic Ports in midline for TEP repair

Metallic ports can be used instead of plastic ports, Stay sutures for 10 mm port, 2(blunt) 5 mm ports below it. Lowest port at least 2-3 cm above pubic bone Carbon dioxide gas is inflated to create the working space.

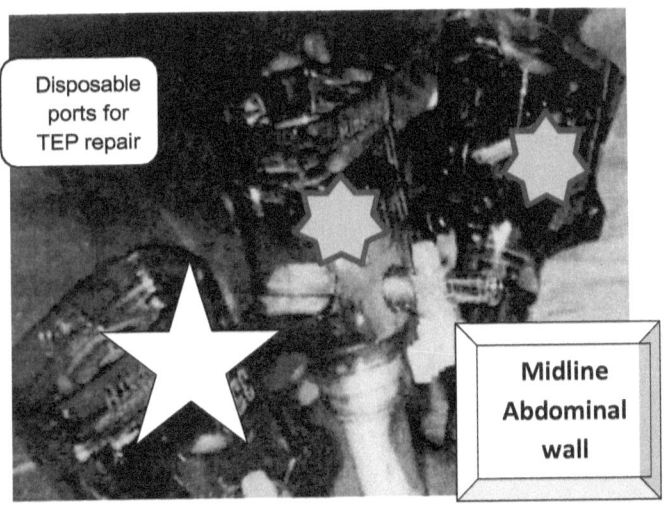

Disposable ports for TEP repair

Midline Abdominal wall

Ports placement method for TEP repair.

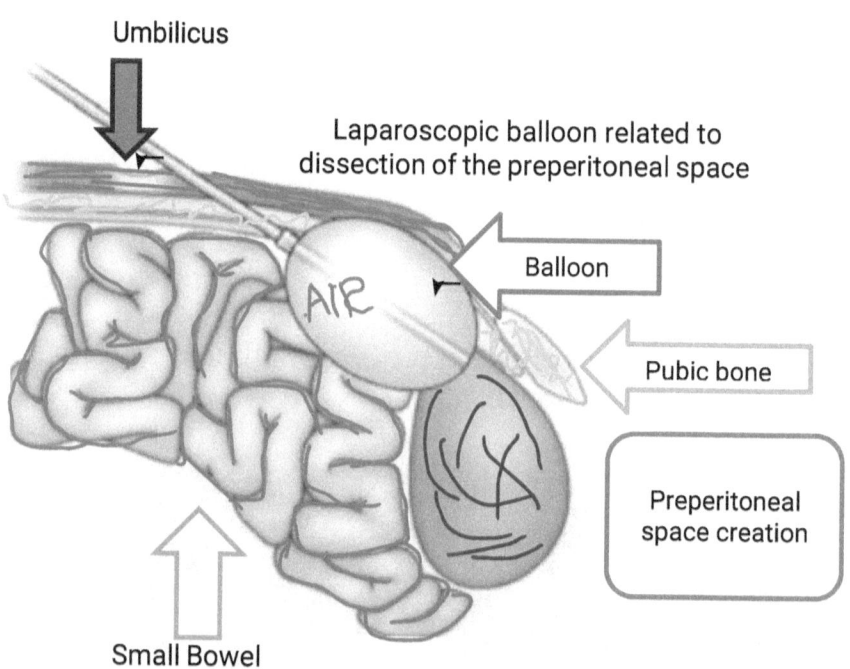

Hernia Anatomy for surgeons and patient awareness

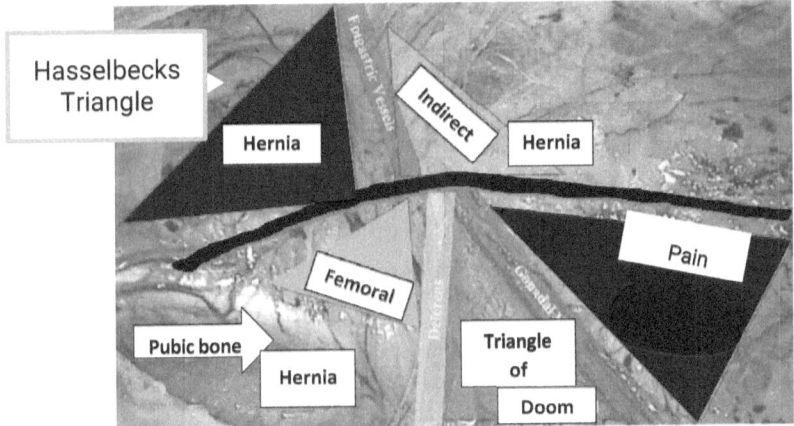

Direct Inguinal hernia
A direct inguinal hernia is protrusion of abdominal contents through the Transversalis fascia within Hesselbach's triangle. The borders of Hesselbach's triangle are the inferior epigastric vessels superolateral, the rectus sheath medially, and inguinal ligament inferiorly.

Indirect Inguinal hernia
An indirect hernia occurs when abdominal contents protrude through the internal inguinal ring and into the inguinal canal. This occurs lateral to the inferior epigastric vessels. The hernia contents may extend into the scrotum.

Femoral hernia
Femoral hernia will present with a characteristic bulge below the inguinal ligament. Strangulation is the most common serious complication of a femoral hernia; these hernias have the highest rate of strangulation (15% to 20%).

Triangle of Doom
The Triangle of Doom is an anatomical triangle defined by the vas deferens medially, gonadal vessel laterally and peritoneum inferiorly. This triangle contains external iliac artery and vein, the deep circumflex iliac vein, the genital branch of genitofemoral nerve and hidden by fascia, the femoral nerve. It bears significance in laparoscopic repair of groin hernia. Surgical staples are avoided here.

Triangle of pain
Similarly, the Triangle of Pain is an important landmark in laparoscopic surgery. The boundaries are: the gonadal vessels (testicular artery and vein) medially, the iliopubic tract superiorly and the peritoneal reflection below. Contents of this triangle include the femoral branch of the genitofemoral nerve, and the Lateral cutaneous nerve of the thigh. After placing the mesh, the surgeon must avoid putting tackers to secure the mesh below the iliopubic tract, or it can injure the nerves. Hence the name 'Triangle of Pain.

Mesh Trimming Technique

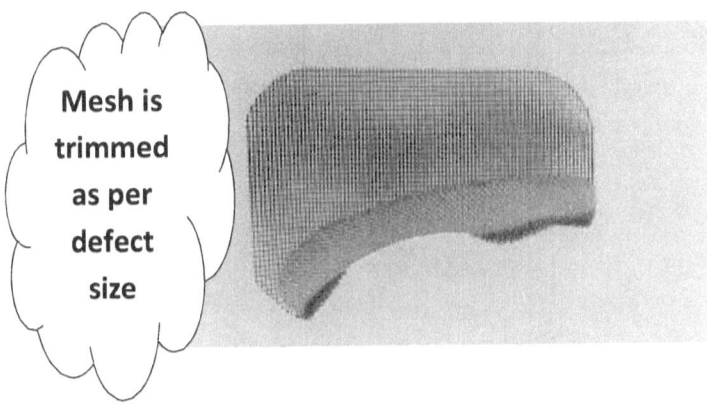

Mesh is trimmed as per defect size

Mesh placement in pre-peritoneal space, mesh acts like a scaffold to strengthen the weakened area without putting tension on surrounding tissues.

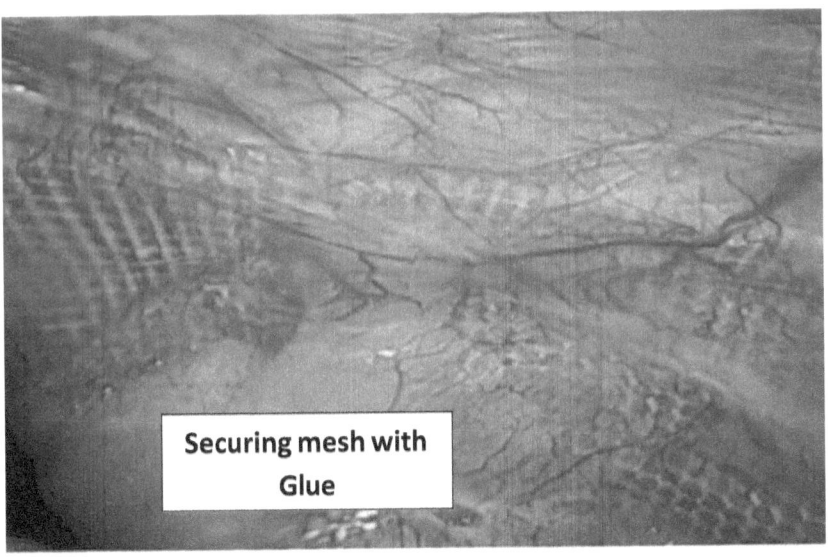

Securing mesh with Glue

Inside Abdominal wall after mesh fixation. / Mesh well integrated into the defect.

Use of glue to secure the mesh in peritoneal space

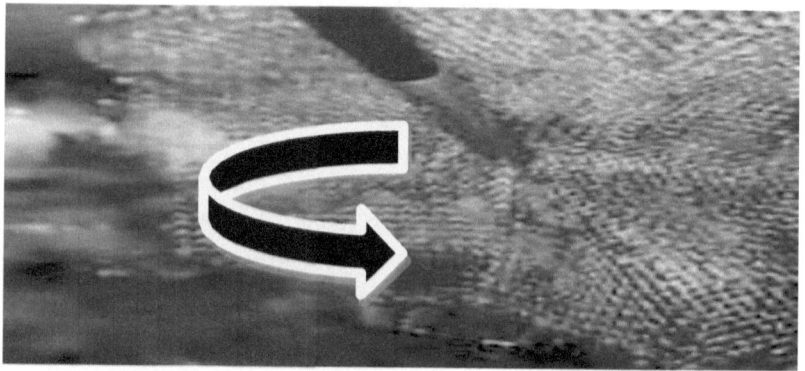

Absorbable or non-absorbable tackers can be used to secure the mesh, Holding the mesh at the time of desufflation helps in keeping it on place.

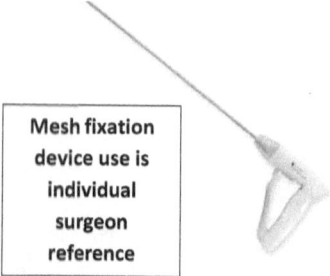

Mesh fixation device use is individual surgeon reference

Tacker's fixation device, tackers can be made up of absorbable or non-absorbable material

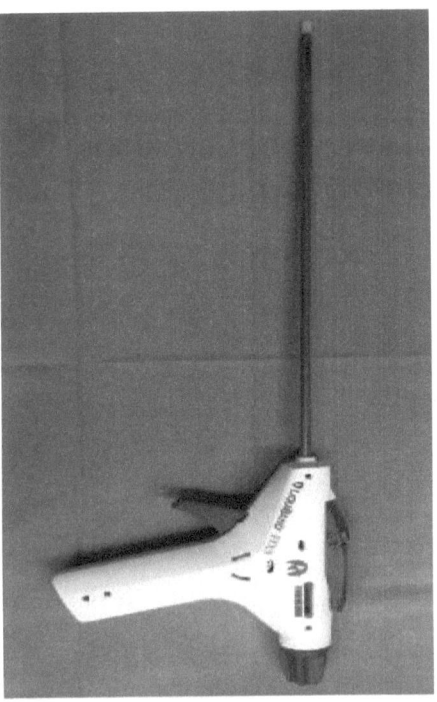

Cyanoacrylate and fibrin glue fixation of mesh have better outcomes with respect to post operative pain. Its cheaper but dries up quickly. Fibrin glue is a biodegradable substance that contains human drive fibrinogen and thrombin activated by calcium chloride.

Complications of TEP Repair

1. **Mesh displacement or erosion into surrounding structures**

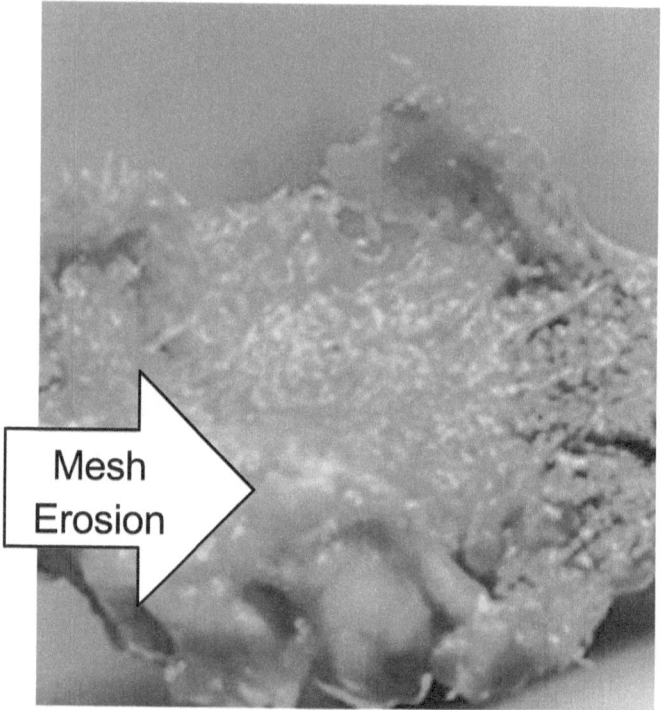

This can be a disastrous complication especially inside the abdomen, in TEP approach the risk of this complication is very low as mesh is placed in pre - peritoneal space.

Mesh migration and erosion is reported in literature, primary migration is associated with inadequate fixation while erosion involves partial disintegration of mesh.

There are isolated incidences of mesh migration to recto-vesical space causing fistula formation with urinary bladder.

2. Seroma or haematoma formation

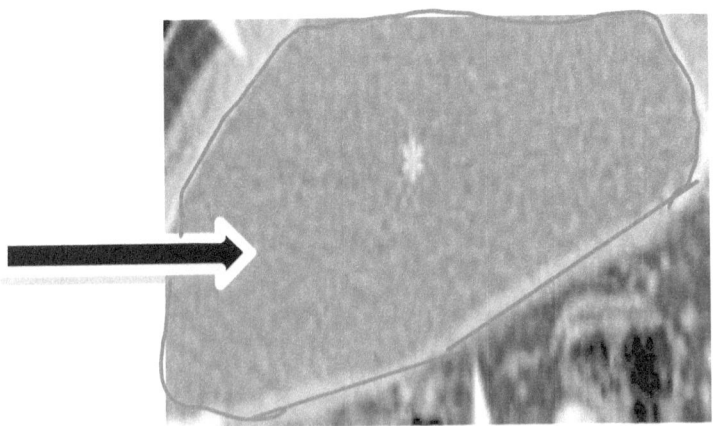

Fluid collection can happen usually sterile, small seromas are managed conservatively without surgical intervention, seroma carries the risk of becoming infected.

3. Infection
Mesh infection risk is 1 in 500 quoted at the time of informed consent process.

4. Recurrence
The risk is 1 in 200 and part of informed consent process.

5. Pain
Pain can occur in up to 5 % patients (1:20).

6. Spermatic cord or vas-deferens injury

Urologist are contacted to repair the vas -deferens if required as this can reduce men fertility the risk is very low otherwise for such injuries, injury to vas deferens can happen after harsh separation of hernial sac.

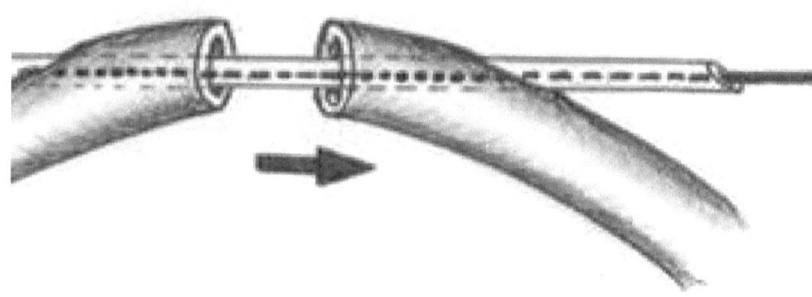

7. Breach of peritoneum and conversion to TAPP or open repair

This is not failure but informed consent from approach need to be changed, advise is informed consent the patient with plus minus proceed for other approaches like open and TAPP (Transabdominal Preperitoneal repair) simultaneously which mean going inside the abdomen to perform the surgery by stripping the peritoneum.

Patient Questions

What is the best method of Hernia Repair?
NICE (National institute of clinical effectiveness) recommend patient to be informed of the risks of open and laparoscopic surgery.

What is the recovery process after hernia repair?
You are expected to go home on same day as a day case surgery until there are some other health issues.

Risks of TEP hernia surgery repair
Majority of patients do not experience any major risks, risks include umbilical wound infection, abdominal wall bruising, surgical emphysema, scrotal and penile bruising.

Hardest Time after Hernia Surgery
it is the discomfort within the first 48 hrs. after the surgery, by the third day after the surgery it usually subsides.

Further Advice
Patients are advised to rest with no weight lifting for 4-6 weeks, laxatives are given to patient at the time of discharge., the surgery is performed in supine position. Risk of any serious complication is 0.5%.

5-10% of patients experience a minor complication. Bladder and vascular injuries are included in the range of serious injuries, some patients can experience debilitating seroma formation.

References

1. Ungureanu CO, Ginghina O, Stanculea F, Iosifescu R, Cristian D, Grigorean VT, Popescu RI, Dobre R, Iordache N. Surgical Outcome in Bilateral Inguinal Hernia Repair: Laparoscopic Total Extraperitoneal Approach (TEP) as Best Approach? Maedica (Bucur). 2023 Dec;18(4):598-606. doi: 10.26574/maedica.2023.18.4.598. PMID: 38348087; PMCID: PMC10859215.

2. Onder T, Altiok M. Do we need mesh fixation at the laparoscopic hernia repair? Asian J Surg. 2023 Oct;46(10):4394-4396. doi: 10.1016/j.asjsur.2023.08.061. Epub 2023 Aug 17. PMID: 37597983.

3. Almutairi H, Alshammari RS, Alharbi MJ, Althobaiti DM, Alghamdi RS, Alsamiri S, Mawash SW, Ahmed DA, Alamoudi AA, Arif FY, Albrahim FM, Alfehaid M, Alanzy HW. Laparoscopic Management of Inguinal Hernia: A Systematic Review and Updated Network Meta-Analysis of Randomized Controlled Trials. Cureus. 2024 Feb 14;16(2):e54192. doi: 10.7759/cureus.54192. PMID: 38496160; PMCID: PMC10942124.

4. Chuah JS, Siow SL, Bujang MA. Quality of life following laparoscopic totally extraperitoneal repair of a unilateral reducible inguinal hernia. Asian J Endosc Surg. 2024 Jul;17(3):e13320. doi: 10.1111/ases.13320. PMID: 38720454.

5. Faye PM, Ndong A, Niasse A, Thiam O, Toure AO, Cisse M. Safety and effectiveness of laparoscopic adult groin hernia repair in Africa: a systematic review and meta-analysis. Hernia. 2024 Apr;28(2):355-365. doi: 10.1007/s10029-023-02931-8. Epub 2024 Feb 7. PMID: 38324087.

www.ingramcontent.com/pod-product-compliance
Lightning Source LLC
Chambersburg PA
CBHW031601210526
45464CB00003B/1379